Living longer:

Maintaining a longer, healthier life shouldn't be too difficult

by

Mary T. Pittman

Table of contents

Chapter 1

Goals for longevity and the three essential factors that contribute to it

- Financial Independence
- Medical care
- Housing
- Purpose, Happiness, and Attitude Are the Three Most Important Elements of a Longevity Lifestyle
- The Quest for Purpose Requires Both Mental and Physical Effort
- The Link Between Having a Purpose in Life and Being Happy
- Lift your spirits by rediscovering the passions that drove you as a child
- Your Choices Will Determine How Long You Live.

Chapter 2

How your level of metabolic fitness influences your likelihood of developing the majority of the chronic diseases that eventually result in death

- What is it About Physical Activity That Is So Amazing?
- The negative health effects of obesity can be mitigated or even reversed via regular exercise.
- Moving Around Can Help Reduce the Pain Associated with Fibromyalgia and Improve Function

Diabetes patients who exercise are better able to control their blood sugar levels

The symptoms of heart disease can be alleviated, and regular exercise can prevent the disease from progressing further

Chapter 3

Why maintaining good metabolic health is essential to living a long and healthy life

Breaking down metabolism

Metabolism vs. 'Metabolic health'

What is it that impacts the metabolism?

How aging changes metabolism

Boost An Aging Metabolism

Conclusions

Chapter 4

Delaying Dementia

Take care of your own heart

Get some exercise and stay active

Participate in pleasurable activities with others

Maintain a balanced and nutritious diet

Engage your mind in some stimulating activity

Chapter 5

the condition of the blood vessels and heart

What exactly is an illness of the heart?

Which symptoms are associated with cardiovascular diseases?

How prevalent is heart disease?

Indicators And Root Causes
What are the reasons for heart disease?
What are the elements that put a person at risk for cardiovascular disease?
What are the signs that someone might have heart disease?
Diagnosis And Tests
How exactly does one go about diagnosing cardiovascular disease?
What kinds of heart disease testing are available to me?
The management as well as treatment of cardiovascular disease
What kind of treatment is there for cardiovascular disease?
Will participating in cardiac rehabilitation make my treatment more effective?
Prevention
How can I protect myself from developing heart disease?
Outlook / Prognosis
What is the prognosis for those who have been diagnosed with cardiovascular disease?
Do I have a higher chance of developing other problems if I have cardiovascular disease?
Living With It
When should I schedule my next visit with my primary care doctor?
Chapter 6
The Importance of Getting Enough Rest

Chapter 7

Consuming foods that promote longevity and health
- This tactic could let you access a lot of opportunities.
- It may be beneficial to your heart
- It may be beneficial to your brain
- It Might Be Beneficial to Your Muscles
- It May Be Beneficial to Your Bones

Chapter 8

The Many Advantages of Exercise
- Is it significant that you sweat?
- The bare essentials

Chapter 9

Increase your level of physical fitness and monitor your improvement

Chapter 10

The importance of muscular power for a long life

Chapter 1

Goals for longevity and the three essential factors that contribute to it

When compared to the other sorts of goals, longevity goals are perhaps the ones with the least amount of intuitiveness. The chance that you will live for a longer period than you anticipate serves as the foundation for your aspirations about longevity.

That is very encouraging, but the retirement income plan you have in place needs to be able to support you throughout those years (unless you intend to make a living playing Pinochle when you are 90).

According to our research, the vast majority of goals related to lifespan may be broken down into the following three categories:

- Financial Independence
- Housing
- Medical Care

Financial Independence

Your longevity has a significant role in determining whether or not you will be able to have a financially secure retirement. It's a good idea to have a plan for your retirement income that allows for 30 years unless your retirement ends up lasting 40 years (which is happening more and more these days).

One of the more challenging aspects of financial planning is figuring out one's life expectancy. We can examine actuarial statistics and calculate with a certain degree of accuracy the dates on which you are likely to pass away, but these predictions are nothing more than statistical estimations.

The most successful users of statistics are huge pension funds and life insurance companies. Because of the large size of the population that these entities cover, they frequently end up appearing to be comparable to historical averages. The actuarial tables might be incorrect by a small margin here and there, but on the whole, they should be able to make a rather accurate forecast of what will occur.

On the other hand, you are not a statistic. There is no way to determine which side of the median life expectancy you will land on when it comes to your lifespan. You are either alive or you are not; there is no such thing as being "basically dead."

And while you are still alive, you need to be able to maintain your standard of living through either a steady salary or a well-diversified investment portfolio. Having said that, the estimations shown here are a good place to start; however, it is important to keep in mind that they are only a beginning place.

Your health and the health of your family should play a significant role in the process of determining how long you want to live. You should undoubtedly make preparations for a lengthy retirement if you are in good health and all of your relatives survived until they were 95 years old. If all of your family members have passed away by the time you reach the age of 75, there is a chance that you won't need to plan for as lengthy of retirement (although under-preparing is a dangerous game to play).

However, none of these things are ever etched into stone. Everyone has heard of folks who smoked two packs of cigarettes each day, drank like a fish, and nevertheless survived well past the age of 100. People who lived a healthy lifestyle participated in regular exercise and ate only the healthiest foods yet managed to pass away in their sixties.

Medical care

Your medical bills are going to get more expensive as you become older, regardless of the length of time you anticipate living. It's common for older folks to rack up greater medical bills, what with trips to the doctor, prescription drugs, mobility aids like walkers, wheelchairs, scooters, and so on. They are also more likely to require long-term care, which can quickly become extremely expensive if it is not adequately planned for.

Housing

It's possible that as you become older, your housing requirements may shift as well. It is the goal of many

individuals to spend their retirement years in the same house they raised their families in, but this is not always achievable. As you get older, you have a wide variety of housing options to choose from; however, they are all rather expensive. And even if you can live in your own house, you could find that you need to make some adjustments to the space so that it can accommodate your requirements.
Your housing requirements in later life are subject to uncertainty, just like everything else. But to tackle these problems, you need to have access to the available resources.

This can suggest that you have a sizable emergency fund that you can tap into to cover any expenses. For other people, it may mean having relatives who are willing to take them in as roommates. There is no one-size-fits-all solution to the challenges of living a long life because each individual's circumstances are unique. You have to determine what it is that works best for you.

Your financial strategy has to take into consideration all of these different scenarios. Even if we have no way of knowing what will take place in the future, we are at least able to speculate intelligently on the various possibilities that are a possibility. You have no idea how long you are going to live or what your latter years will be like, but you do know that you will have to provide for others who are dependent on you in some way. The objective is to get to a point where you are confident that you will have the resources necessary to overcome any difficulties that come your way.

Purpose, Happiness, and Attitude Are the Three Most Important Elements of a Longevity Lifestyle

Having a reason to get up in the morning is one of the most important factors in determining your health and lifespan. Some people believe that having a sense of direction and broad goals, or even particular ones, such as learning a new language or playing an instrument like the piano or guitar, is essential to having a purpose in life.

When I think of purpose, I think of making an effort toward doing things that are meaningful to you and having daily goals that are attainable and within your control. In the end, it is up to you to determine the things that give your life meaning. To give you an example, if gardening has become a passion of yours, then giving it a sense of purpose in your life would lead you to read gardening books, talk to neighbors about what they're planting and share ideas and tips, speak to professionals at nurseries, and move things around in your yard to improve and enhance their health and visual impact. You are getting the point.

Your time, attention, and even the relationships in your life can be better organized when you have a sense of purpose. It is much simpler to force yourself out of bed and get moving once you realize that you need to get up and get moving to start making phone calls and arranging for a community event in which you are participating.

People who have ambitions for their lives and strive toward achieving those ambitions are more likely to experience feelings of self-worth and fulfillment, which in turn enables them to keep a positive attitude in life. Finding a sense of purpose early in life has been shown to improve overall health, but I believe that finding a renewed sense of purpose is what propels people into thriving later in life. Find a new way to cook if you've been doing the same thing for a long time and find yourself getting bored with it. If cooking doesn't excite you anymore, try another hobby or activity. If you live to be 100 or older, you will have multiple lifetime's worths of goals and aspirations to pursue if you make it that far.

If you are unsure whether or not purpose and lifespan are connected, think about this. Research has shown that contrary to popular belief, living in the White House does not result in an early onset of aging for the President of the United States.

According to research published in 2011 by S. Jay Olshansky, Ph.D., at the University of Illinois at Chicago, the average lifespan of a US President for the past half-century has been between 8 12, and 9 years longer than that of the typical American.

These individuals had what is commonly referred to as the most demanding job in the world, and it is well-established that prolonged exposure to high amounts of stress can hasten one's mortality. Then, why do so many former presidents go on to live such long lives after leaving office?

It's possible that the fact that these men's lives were driven by purpose, and that they were rewarded and praised for their hard work, is the thing that ties them together. In addition, after their terms in office were over, they continued to be driven by a sense of purpose and a desire to make a difference in the world.

The Quest for Purpose Requires Both Mental and Physical Effort

In 2015, at the age of 105, Hidekichi Miyazaki, a Japanese grandfather of ten and father of four, raced the 100-meter dash in 42.22 seconds. He set a world record for an athlete of his age. In the sport of track and field, he broke a record for the Guinness Book of World Records by becoming the oldest competitive sprinter. At the Kyoto Masters Tournament, he not only competed in the discus but also in the shot put.

It wasn't his competitive running or his race times that struck me as being the most interesting aspect of his life. It was his awareness of the bigger picture. In the 33 years leading up to the moment when he decided to start competing in track and field at the ripe old age of 93, he honed his skills as a calligrapher and spent time with his pals playing Japanese chess. For several years, those routines provided him with both purpose and friendship. However, as his buddies began to pass away due to old age, he wanted to find something that he could do by himself; this is how the track and field events came about.

Miyazaki is vigilant about his training. His daughter claims that he goes to the park nearby for his workouts daily, except when it's raining. His normal workout consists of a one hundred-meter dash followed by three sets of shotput to practice.
He has no intention of "taking it easy," and he has established a new objective for himself to cut his sprint time of 42.22 seconds down to 36 or even 35 seconds.

His narrative demonstrates that one must put in some effort, whether cerebral or physical, to find one's true calling and the enjoyment it brings; one must expand both their intellect and their body.

The Link Between Having a Purpose in Life and Being Happy

The intelligent doctor Becky Su, who practices both Western and Chinese medicine, has some words of advice to share with the world: "Happiness is contagious. If you can be a source of happiness and joy for only one night, then by the time the night is over, everyone who has been in your presence will have experienced happiness. Even when things are difficult, there are still opportunities for joy, and this is a good reminder of that fact. In the same way that there is no limit to the quantity of love that may exist, there is no limit to the amount of happiness that can exist in the world.

When she talks about happiness, Dr. Su is probably at her most motivating and useful. Her three strategies for achieving happiness are both straightforward and in-depth:

An old proverb advises, "If you can't change it, don't think about it," and this is sound advice. Do not lose any sleep over the fact that your adult child is having difficulty if it is something that you are unable to change. Take care of your health so that you can be there for the people who need you.

"You must first permit yourself before you can allow others to enjoy delight. You can't force yourself to be happy, but you can permit yourself to choose happiness for yourself.

"Maintain your focus on things that are beautiful and worthy of admiration. Your brain is capable of being trained. Your disposition, your way of thinking, the way you feel right now, and the way you will feel tomorrow are not set in stone. We are hardwired to recognize when something is wrong since it is a survival mechanism, but we can work against this instinct. Can the monk move the mountain? is a question that is often posed by Chinese thinkers. The question that must be answered is, "Which point of view do you want to investigate?"

To strive for happiness as a goal to improve the overall quality of our life is without a doubt an admirable endeavor. But the entire area of happiness research is revealing that being happy isn't just a "bonus" for living a good life; happiness may help us live longer, inspire healthier habits, and even change our DNA.

In this sense, happiness does not entail always having a positive attitude or acting in a Pollyannaish manner. The goal is not to achieve perfection or to do everything just properly to be completely content all the time. There are times when one is happy, but there are also times when one is sad or grieving. Maintaining a steadfast commitment to the "proper" behaviors, including the routines that I talk about in my blogs, does not ensure a long life, and pursuing correctness at the expense of joy results in a life that is only partially lived. The ability to view and engage with the world in a manner that is characterized by optimism, a feeling of purpose, and an energizing spark of life that may be contagious is at the heart of happiness.

Lift your spirits by rediscovering the passions that drove you as a child

When it comes to living a long and healthy life, our attitudes matter a great deal. It has been demonstrated that if a person believes that they look and feel younger than their actual biological age, they are more likely to live longer than another individual who feels their age or even older than that. According to the findings of Becca Levy, Ph.D., a researcher on aging at the Yale School of Public Health, having a positive attitude toward becoming older will help you live an additional 7.5 years on average. Whether we conceive of it in terms of limitations and inevitable decline or of lifelong possibility and living at the edge of our capabilities, our views about aging impact how we feel about our health.

My research has led me to the conclusion that those individuals who enjoy a longer and more fulfilled life span are more likely to keep some form of totem that serves as a link to their earlier selves. There was a resident who was around 90 years old and yet enjoyed riding the Ferris wheel every year.

However, it appears that the contrary is also true. People who believe they are "too old" to participate in some activities that they might otherwise enjoy or who believe that they are expected to "look and act their age" appear to age before their time.

Your Choices Will Determine How Long You Live.

Wellness Warriors, if you believe that getting older means becoming less active or that you are "over the hill," you are less likely to take care of yourself. You'll give in to decline. If you believe that the way you feel dictates how old you are, you will be more inclined to engage in good behaviors, which will result in longer and healthier life. You will eat foods that nourish your body rather than foods that harm it. You will have the opportunity to receive the restorative sleep you require, which will allow you to maintain your energy levels throughout the day. You'll move more and sit less.

Because of all of these behaviors, you will not only start to feel better, but you will also start to feel younger. This, in turn, will help you have the best possible health for the rest of your life.

Chapter 2

How your level of metabolic fitness influences your likelihood of developing the majority of the chronic diseases that eventually result in death

When everything is considered, chronic diseases are the greatest cause of death and the major cause of disability in the United States. According to the Centers for Disease Control and Prevention, six out of ten American individuals have at least one chronic disease, and four out of ten have two or more chronic diseases.

It is important to know that exercise can play a role in managing problems and symptoms that you may already be experiencing. Bradley Prigge, a wellness exercise specialist at the Mayo Clinic Healthy Living Program, says that exercise can play a role in managing problems and symptoms that you may already be experiencing. This is something that health experts regularly claim is one of the top things you can do to lower your risk of developing one of these chronic problems in the first place.

"If you look at a range of things like high blood pressure, high cholesterol levels, persistent pain, and inflammation — all of these things that are risk factors and symptoms of various chronic conditions — across the board, there is a huge value that comes from increasing your level of fitness and your level of physical activity in your life," says Prigge. "When you consider several factors, including high blood pressure, high cholesterol, chronic pain, and inflammation, all of which are risk factors and symptoms of various chronic diseases

For instance, aerobic exercise can aid in the prevention of heart disease. However, if you already have signs of heart problems, such as high cholesterol or high blood pressure, moderate-intensity exercise can aid in preventing such problems from progressing into more serious ones (such as heart attack or stroke).

Strength training helps build muscle and promotes healthy joints, which allows healthy persons to maintain their range of motion and function as they get older. On the other hand, this kind of exercise can assist patients with type 2 diabetes in better controlling their glucose levels and reducing the discomfort associated with arthritis. Simple flexibility exercises can assist enhance a joint's range of motion, which in turn reduces the risk of falling for everyone. persons who suffer from arthritis will find that stretching helps reduce joint discomfort and keeps it from becoming worse.

What is it About Physical Activity That Is So Amazing?

According to Shawn Flanagan, Ph.D., an assistant professor in the department of sports medicine and nutrition at the University of Pittsburgh, exercise is considered to be "pleiotropic," which is a scientific term that simply means that it has "many impacts." According to him, regular exercise can improve sleep quality, safeguard and boost brain function, cultivate or preserve bone, and muscle, and promote a healthy immune system, heart, and other connective tissues.

According to Dr. Flanagan, depending on the situation, "wounds heal faster, medication doses can sometimes be reduced or maintained, and disease severity can be improved dramatically." The implications of these benefits are significant.

"Exercise increases the release of several substances that protect neurons, facilitate recovery from injury, and presumably strengthen the integrity of the blood-brain barrier," says Flanagan about the effects exercise has on the brain. The blood-brain barrier is a collection of blood vessels that regulates what is carried from the blood into the brain. This barrier ensures that harmful substances, viruses, and inflammation are kept out of the brain while allowing beneficial cells and molecules to get through.

According to Flanagan's explanation, all of these factors are significant when it comes to warding off chronic disease. Damage to neurons and inflammation in the brain, for instance, are known to occur in patients who suffer from neurological conditions such as multiple sclerosis, Alzheimer's disease, and Parkinson's disease, for instance.

According to Scott Parker, a personal trainer in private practice in Los Angeles who is also a representative for the American Heart Association, "exercise may help" with any ailment that exists. People tend to overlook the fact that one of the primary purposes of exercise is to maintain and improve our overall health, even though there is a lot of discussion about how to exercise to obtain a certain body type or look.

A closer look at how exercise can improve the management of numerous chronic health disorders and provide symptom alleviation is presented here. Also, keep in mind that if you have a chronic health condition or other chronic symptoms, you should consult your physician before beginning a new fitness regimen to ensure that it is safe for you to undertake and that it will not cause any additional damage to your body.

The negative health effects of obesity can be mitigated or even reversed via regular exercise.

Increasing one's level of physical activity can be beneficial in the fight against obesity for a few different reasons. Obesity is a dangerous chronic condition that affects more than four in ten persons in the United States, which translates to a prevalence rate of 42.4 percent. A body mass index (BMI) of 30 or more is considered obese. In addition, the obesity rate among children in the United States is approximately 19.3 percent. There are an estimated 112,000 deaths that can be prevented each year that are attributed to obesity, and this number is growing. The percentage of adults in this country who were classified obese in 1980 was 13.4 percent, which is 29 percent less than the current number. the

According to Parker, "I think that number one, a huge difficulty is that the vast majority of people do not regard obesity as a chronic disease, but it is."

And moving around is one of the first things you can do to prevent some of the negative impacts of being overweight, such as having high cholesterol and high blood pressure, both of which can increase the risk of hypertension and cardiovascular disease. According to Parker, it is not about getting "slim" or "getting abs;" rather, the focus should be on being healthy. Any increase in physical activity, even something as simple as walking a few more kilometers a day or riding a bike, can go a long way toward helping you achieve a healthier weight.

According to research that was published in August 2019, exercising can help people who are obese reduce their chance of acquiring a variety of ailments, including heart disease, type 2 diabetes, some malignancies, depression, anxiety, and others.

Exercising will assist you in reducing weight, which is a necessary component of the treatment plan recommended for the vast majority of obese patients.
And according to review research that was published in 2021 in the journal iScience, increased fitness and physical activity is associated with a longer life even if you don't weigh more in people who are obese. This was shown in the study of obese persons.

Moving Around Can Help Reduce the Pain Associated with Fibromyalgia and Improve Function

If you are one of the four million adults in the United States who have been diagnosed with fibromyalgia, you may suffer from significant chronic pain across your entire body, exhaustion, headaches, trouble sleeping, and depression.

People who are living with this constant agony, which can at times be all-consuming, may find that exercising is a method to make them feel better about themselves. Aerobic exercises, weight training, stretching, and balancing training, for example, have all been demonstrated to help lessen the pain and handicap associated with the illness.

An aerobic exercise intervention was found to improve the overall quality of life by reducing the intensity of pain, improving physical function, and reducing stiffness and fatigue in 839 adults diagnosed with fibromyalgia, according to a review that was published in 2017 in the Cochrane Database of Systematic Reviews. The review analyzed data from 13 clinical trials that were conducted in which the participants had fibromyalgia.

Another study found that practicing qigong, a traditional Chinese system of exercises and breathing, for 30 to 45 minutes each day for six to eight weeks not only helped people's physical and mental health but also eased people's chronic pain and helped them sleep better. The findings of this study were published in the issue of the journal Medicines which was published in June 2017.

Diabetes patients who exercise are better able to control their blood sugar levels

Regular exercise is an important lifestyle intervention that can help people with diabetes manage their illness and prevent further complications that may result from it. In the US, 34.2 million people suffer from diabetes.

Physical activity has been shown to improve insulin sensitivity, which is the ability of the hormone to do its job, which is to lower your blood sugar levels. Not only can regular exercise help you lose weight, but it can also help you better control your glucose levels in people who have type 2 diabetes.

More effective management of glucose, an increase in insulin sensitivity, and a reduction in overall body mass all contribute to the prevention of complications that are closely associated with diabetes. These complications include hypertension, heart disease, and high blood pressure.

In 2010, the American Diabetes Association and the American College of Sports Medicine issued a joint statement in which they recommended that patients with type 2 diabetes engage in regular physical activity to assist control the condition. This recommendation was included in the statement.

The symptoms of heart disease can be alleviated, and regular exercise can prevent the disease from progressing further

The prevention and treatment of heart disease, which is the leading cause of death in the United States each year, can be significantly aided by regular exercise.

The American Heart Association published a report in 2018 that examined the relationship between physical exercise and its impact on the prevention and treatment of coronary artery disease (CAD). According to the findings of the study, regular participation in structured exercise training, which involves incorporating a fitness or exercise routine into one's daily life, can help reduce the symptoms of coronary artery disease (CAD), improve blood flow in the heart, and reduce the risk of death. According to the findings of the research, the enhanced oxygen circulation that results from exercising in a way that improves blood flow helps to avoid the kind of plaque formation in the arteries that lead to difficulties caused by coronary artery disease (CAD).

According to Prigge, physical activity is one of the most important factors in the battle against heart disease. If the idea of going to the gym makes you feel like you're being punished, Parker suggests that you try going on a walk, riding a bike, or performing simple aerobic exercises in your living room instead. Any one of these options could be beneficial.

If you are beginning a new fitness program and have risk factors for heart disease, it is important to note that the intensity level should not be increased too rapidly. Always to your primary care physician before beginning a new routine. And if you already have heart disease and you start feeling chest pains, dizziness, irregular heartbeats, or shortness of breath for no apparent reason, then it is necessary to take a break and let your doctor know about the particular symptoms you are having. If you already have heart disease, even a mild form of the condition, certain types of exercise may make your symptoms worse and may not be safe for you to do.

Even if you don't have a chronic condition, regular exercise can help you age healthily.

Exercising is beneficial for bodies in general, which is one of the reasons why it is beneficial for bodies that already have chronic diseases. Exercise helps all bodies. According to several studies, maintaining a healthy level of physical fitness can assist in delaying the aging process.

At the level of individual cells, high-intensity aerobic exercise was shown to be capable, according to the findings of a study that was carried out in March 2017 and published in the journal Cell Metabolism, of reversing some of the indications of aging.

High-intensity aerobic workouts did improve a person's aerobic capacity (that is, lung function), as well as the mitochondrial function of skeletal muscles. However, working out won't turn back the clock (declining mitochondrial function is associated with muscle wasting and muscle loss in the elderly).

According to Flanagan, all of us need to maintain an active lifestyle as we become older. The major objective is to keep up the activity level.

Flanagan recommends seeing a medical professional determine whether or not the duration, frequency, and intensity of your workouts are acceptable for your needs. Do, however, make it a point to experiment with a wide range of different kinds of physical activity, such as high-intensity exercise and resistance or strength training. According to Flanagan, the most effective technique to preserve one's muscle mass and strength is to engage in resistance training.

According to Prigge, it is normal to be concerned about how the natural process of aging can slow you down or restrict the things you can perform. Your best protection against that is to work out regularly and maintain a physically active lifestyle. "It enables you to carry out activities that you might have previously taken for granted, he adds."It's something that you might have taken for granted." "[Getting regular exercise] helps you experience more in life," which is a benefit of exercising regularly.

Chapter 3

Why maintaining good metabolic health is essential to living a long and healthy life

You've probably encountered someone with a "quick metabolism," or perhaps you are that person yourself. People with fast metabolisms appear to be able to eat everything they want without gaining even an ounce of fat from doing so. Metabolism is a topic that receives a lot of attention, particularly in connection with weight loss. Maintaining a healthy metabolism is not only crucial for controlling one's weight and maintaining good body composition, but it is also important for maximizing one's healthspan and lifespan. Current research has discovered that having a metabolism that is "youthful" is a powerful predictor of both the absence of disease and the length of one's lifespan. One of the most crucial aspects of healthy aging is having a good understanding of what metabolism is and how to keep it up.

Breaking down metabolism

The collective name for the series of biological reactions that take place in each cell of our body is called metabolism.
Food is the primary means by which we take in nutrients; it consists of carbohydrate, protein, and fat components. During the process of digestion, these macronutrients are broken down into smaller, simpler molecules. In particular, amino acids are derived from proteins, simple sugars are derived from carbs, and glycerol and free fatty acids are derived from fats (from lipids). These "building blocks" are essential for the formation of cellular structures and the delivery of energy throughout our bodies. This "energy" is supplied in the form of a molecule known as adenosine triphosphate (ATP).

How many calories you burn each day is one way to think about your metabolism, which is sometimes referred to as your "total energy expenditure." The three basic components that make up a person's total energy expenditure are their basal metabolic rate (BMR), their total energy expenditure from physical activity, and their total energy expenditure from diet-induced thermogenesis. The basal metabolic rate, or BMR, is the amount of energy that must be expended at rest for us to continue living and for biological processes to be maintained. The amount of energy we expend while at rest accounts for around 60–70% of our overall energy consumption. Consuming food requires us to expend a certain amount of energy to digest it, absorb it, and store it. This quantity of energy is referred to as diet-induced thermogenesis or diet-induced energy expenditure. This component accounts for anywhere between 5 and 10 percent of the overall energy expenditure. The final component of total energy expenditure is the one that varies the greatest from year to year and accounts for anywhere between 20 and 40 percent of total energy expenditure. This is what we mean when we talk about our "energy expenditure" when we talk about physical activity. This includes the energy that we consume for both exercise and everyday activity.

Metabolism vs. 'Metabolic health'

The term "metabolic health" can be used to refer to metabolism in a more general sense. However, one way to think about metabolism is the process of burning calories. The word "metabolic health" is often misunderstood, although in general, having "optimal" levels of blood sugar, cholesterol, and blood pressure, as well as having a healthy body composition, is considered to be "metabolically healthy." This term is sometimes abused and confusing. Even this can be somewhat complicated because there is probably not a single "perfect" for any of these components; rather, there is only what is "optimal" for each specific person.

If our metabolism is in good shape, it indicates that our bodies can make efficient use of the nutrients that we take in and produce the energy that we require. It means that our organ systems perform "optimally" for what we require at all phases of life and that we have healthy mitochondria, which are factories that produce energy and are finely calibrated. Just "burning calories" is not nearly as crucial as maintaining a healthy metabolism, which is of course much more vital. It is essential to have optimal metabolic health to age in a healthy manner and live a long life.

What is it that impacts the metabolism?

The first, second, and third primary aspects of metabolism have already been described. These three aspects are additionally impacted by a plethora of lifestyle, environmental, and genetic factors, all of which have the potential to modify how our bodies process nutrients and make use of energy.

Genetics: Decades of research have uncovered evidence suggesting that genetics have a role in determining how much energy (calories) we use throughout a typical day. The qualities that we inherit could be responsible for as much as forty percent of the variation in total energy consumption.

Composition of the diet It's possible that the food we consume is just as crucial to our metabolism as the amount of food we eat. According to the findings of certain studies, meals that are high in protein lead to a higher rate of energy expenditure. This is because protein requires more energy to digest and process than a comparable amount of carbohydrates or fat. In reality, each macronutrient contributes a unique amount of the type of energy that is necessary for the digestive processes. When expressed as a percentage of the calories provided by each macronutrient, the amount of energy required to digest and absorb fat is 0–3 percent, whereas the amount of energy required for carbohydrates is 5–10 percent, and the amount of energy required for protein is 20–30 percent. This indicates that we burn approximately.25 calories for every gram of fat, 1 calorie for every gram of carbohydrates, and between 2 and 3 calories for every gram of protein that we consume.

You may believe that those who engage in regular physical exercise have a higher resting metabolic rate than individuals who do not engage in regular physical activity, however, this may not be the case. Even if exercise training causes an increase in total energy expenditure since it leads to a higher level of physical activity, it might not impact the amount of energy that is expended while at rest. On the other hand, certain types of exercise, such as high-intensity interval training (HIIT), will keep your metabolic rate elevated for some time after the workout is finished. This means that you will have a higher rate of calorie burn throughout the day.

Muscle mass: Because of the demand for energy to power our muscles, having more muscle mass results in an increase in the amount of energy that is required by the body. People who have a larger percentage of their body that is made up of lean mass burn more calories at rest. In addition, having more muscle mass makes it easier to regulate levels of glucose and insulin in the blood, which ultimately results in improved metabolic health.

Hormones: Hormones can affect both the amount of energy that we utilize and the efficiency with which we use it. Leptin and ghrelin, which are referred to as "hunger hormones," along with insulin, can control the amount of energy we take in and how efficiently we use glucose. Additionally, thyroid hormones control the amount of energy expended by the body by regulating temperature, growth processes, and the metabolism of glucose and fat. The natural decline in thyroid hormone levels that occurs with aging may be one factor that contributes to a slower metabolism and a relative rise in body fat.

How aging changes metabolism

The amount of energy we expend while at rest decreases with age by approximately 1-2 percent each decade.
This could suggest that between the ages of 20 and 70, your body's ability to burn energy decreases by approximately 400 calories every day. What might be the cause of this?

A decrease in total muscle mass is one of the causes. If you lose muscle, which is a significant source of energy consumption, this will result in a decrease in your overall metabolic rate. Additionally, as we get older, our fat mass goes up, which leads to adverse changes in our body composition. Because fat uses less energy than muscle does, this results in a decrease in the amount of energy that is expended while at rest. It is possible that muscle is not the only tissue that deteriorates with age; in fact, some investigations have indicated that the metabolic rate of certain organs also decreases with age.

Along with a shift in body composition, overall physical activity levels are often lower in persons as they age. In old age, one's tendency to be "less active" contributes to a reduction in the amount of energy expended as a result of the physical activity caused by exercise and general movements.

As we become older, how we get our energy from food sources also alters. There is a correlation between being older and having decreased insulin sensitivity, glucose absorption, and fat oxidation. Our mitochondria and other pathways that produce energy become less efficient at taking in and utilizing fuel sources as we age. Studies have revealed that aging causes a decrease in the mitochondria's ability to oxidize glucose and fat, as well as an inability of the mitochondria to "switch" between using glucose and fat as fuel sources. This phenomenon is referred to as "metabolic flexibility."

Boost An Aging Metabolism

It is believed that metabolic dysfunction and energy dysregulation lead to a more rapid aging process as well as a worse quality of life in individuals. It is feasible, thankfully, to revitalize a metabolism that has slowed down and become less effective by making adjustments to one's lifestyle.

Exercising regularly is one of the most effective ways for people of any age to enhance their metabolic health. It's possible that lifting weights is the answer! Strength training increases muscle strength and power, as well as produces lean muscle mass that helps the body burn more calories. The capacity of mitochondria can be increased, insulin sensitivity can be improved, and overall metabolic function can be boosted by the practice of aerobic endurance exercise, sometimes known as "cardio." It is possible to maintain a high rate of energy expenditure and improve metabolic flexibility by adhering to a regular exercise plan that includes both resistance training and aerobic exercise and that is performed multiple times per week.

The phrase "intermittent fasting" (IF) refers to a method of eating less often than usual. The consumption of fatty acids and ketones for energy production helps promote a "metabolic switch" away from the utilization of carbohydrates as a source of energy during a fast. This can assist in building the metabolic machinery necessary for effectively burning fat and glucose. Both intermittent fasting (such as the 5:2 diet) and daily time-restricted feeding (also known as TRF) are fasting regimens that have been supported by scientific research and are used to encourage metabolic switching and to keep metabolic flexibility.

Increase your intake of protein: Consuming a greater amount of protein may be essential to forestall the consequences of a natural decrease in muscle mass that occurs with advancing age. To maximize the amount of muscle protein synthesis that occurs after exercise, consuming forty grams of protein is recommended. That's somewhere between six and eight ounces of meat. Eat a sufficient quantity of protein at each meal throughout the day, and consider taking an amino acid supplement containing leucine (or eating foods rich in leucine, such as meat and cheese), because leucine is an amino acid that stimulates protein synthesis by activating the Mechanistic Target of Rapamycin (mTOR). The single most effective way to achieve maximum stimulation of muscle protein synthesis is to combine resistance training with a meal that is high in protein.

Enter ketosis: Because there are fewer carbohydrates available, ketogenic and low-carb, high-fat diets encourage metabolic flipping by compelling the body to convert to using fatty acids and ketones for energy rather than carbohydrates. The ability to utilize fat and ketone bodies ensures that there is sufficient energy available to all of the body's tissues, which is especially important as we age and glucose metabolism slows down, which can contribute to neurodegeneration. Ketosis can be induced without the use of a low-carb diet or fasting by taking exogenous ketone supplements or drinking ketone-containing beverages. This method was just recently found. By increasing metabolic switching, exogenous ketones can help increase healthspan, and they may even be able to offset the effects of aging on memory performance.

Conclusions

The natural progression of aging does not necessarily have to be accompanied by slowing metabolism. It is possible to achieve healthy and successful metabolic aging by managing your health through nutrition, exercise, and ongoing participation in both physical and cognitive activities. The secret to a long and fruitful life is maintaining a healthy metabolism. And fortunately, most of it is under your control.

Chapter 4

Delaying Dementia

There is currently no cure for dementia, even though scientists are making significant progress in researching therapies for the condition. While medications can treat some of the effects of the underlying disease, other therapies help manage the symptoms of the condition.

Taking action in the five areas that are discussed below may help lower the risk of acquiring dementia and postpone the beginning of the condition.

Take care of your own heart

Particularly reducing the impact of vascular dementia can be accomplished by exercising proper control over blood pressure, cholesterol levels, Type II diabetes, and obesity. Quitting smoking is another factor that fits under this category; doing so reduces the number of neurotoxins in the body, which helps prevent additional damage to neurons.

Get some exercise and stay active

It is believed that physical activity might stimulate the brain to create new neurons, so slowing the progression of cognitive loss. Activities that help build muscle also contribute to improved balance (reducing falls). Exercising not only lifts your mood but also helps protect your heart by lowering the risk factors that are related to cardiovascular disease.

Participate in pleasurable activities with others

Participating in social activities not only boosts cerebral activity but also strengthens emotional connections to others and the neural networks that underlie memory. Isolation from one's social circle raises one's probability of developing dementia and also raises one's probability of developing hypertension, depression, and coronary heart disease, all of which are also risk factors for dementia.

Maintain a balanced and nutritious diet

The consumption of a diet rich in fruits, vegetables, legumes, and nuts; the substitution of butter for olive oil; the consumption of fish at least twice per week; the addition of herbs and spices in place of salt; and the restriction of red meat have all been shown in research to be associated with a lower risk of developing dementia. There is a correlation between consuming processed foods that are high in fat and trans fat and an increased risk of dementia.

Engage your mind in some stimulating activity

The principle of "use it or lose it" is central to this discussion. Engaging your brain in novel activities that stretch its capabilities will help develop new brain cells and enhance connections in the existing ones. It's possible that they won't have any effect on memory, but there is some evidence that they help with executive functions like decision-making and reasoning, and that they also help things get processed more quickly.

Chapter 5

the condition of the blood vessels and heart

What exactly is an illness of the heart?

The term "cardiovascular disease" (sometimes known as "heart disease") refers to a set of conditions that affect the cardiovascular system, specifically the heart and blood arteries. These conditions can damage your blood vessels as well as one or more parts of your heart, including the entire heart. Depending on their status, a person may show symptoms of a disease or may not show any symptoms at all (not feel anything at all).

Problems with the following organs or blood vessels are included in the category of heart disease:

- Abnormal rhythms of the heart
- Heart valve disease.
- Plaque buildup can cause a narrowing of the blood arteries in your heart as well as in other organs and throughout your body.
- Stress on the heart and difficulty relaxing are symptoms.

- Congenital heart and blood vascular conditions are present from birth.
- Having issues with the outer lining of your heart.

Which symptoms are associated with cardiovascular diseases?

There are a wide variety of cardiovascular diseases, some of which include but are not limited to the following:

- A problem with the electrical conduction system of the heart, also known as arrhythmia, is a condition that can cause abnormal cardiac rhythms or pulse rates.
- Valve disease is a problem with your heart's valves, which are structures that allow blood to pass from one chamber to another chamber or blood channel. Symptoms of valve disease include tightening of the valves or leaking of the valves.
- A problem with the blood vessels of your heart, such as blockages, is referred to as coronary artery disease (CAD).
- Fluid buildup and shortness of breath are symptoms of heart failure, which is caused by problems with the pumping and relaxing functions of the heart.
- A problem with the blood vessels in your arms, legs, or abdominal organs, such as narrowing or blockages, is referred to as peripheral arterial disease (PAD).
- Aortic disease is a problem with the big blood vessel that transports blood from the heart to the brain and

the rest of the body. Symptoms of the aortic disease include dilatation of the blood vessel and aneurysm of the blood vessel.

- The term "congenital heart disease" refers to an issue with the heart that is present at birth and can affect various areas of the organ.
- Diseases that affect the pericardium, or the lining of the heart, such as pericarditis and pericardial effusion, are collectively referred to as pericardial diseases.
- Diseases of the blood vessels that supply blood to the brain are referred to as cerebrovascular diseases. These diseases can cause the blood vessels to become constricted or blocked.
- A blockage in the veins or blood arteries that carry blood from the brain and the rest of the body back to the heart is known as deep vein thrombosis.

How prevalent is heart disease?

The United States and the rest of the globe both rank cardiovascular disease as the main cause of mortality. Heart disease claims the lives of 655,000 people in the United States every year.

In the United States, about half of all individuals suffer from at least one form of cardiovascular disease. Men and women are both impacted by it. For women, cardiovascular disease is the main cause of death. It does not discriminate based on age, race, or financial status; it affects people of all three.

Indicators And Root Causes

What are the reasons for heart disease?

There are many different types of cardiovascular disease, each with its unique risk factors and risk factors for complications. For instance, coronary artery disease and peripheral artery disease are both brought on by atherosclerosis, also known as the development of plaque in the arteries. Arrhythmias can be brought on by coronary artery disease, scarring of the heart muscle, genetic issues, or adverse reactions to drugs. Inflammatory valve disease can be caused by aging, infections, or rheumatic disease.

What are the elements that put a person at risk for cardiovascular disease?

If you have risk factors such as those listed below, your likelihood of developing the cardiovascular disease may be higher.

- Unhealthy levels of blood pressure (hypertension).
- Poor cholesterol management (hyperlipidemia)
- Tobacco usage.
- Diabetes.
- a family history of cardiac illness.
- A sedentary way of life or becoming obese.
- Consumption of a lot of sodium, sugar, and fat in one's diet.
- Consumption of alcohol in excess.

- Preeclampsia or toxemia.
- Diabetes mellitus in pregnancy
- Conditions characterized by persistent inflammation or autoimmunity.
- Kidney illness that persists over time

What are the signs that someone might have heart disease?

The symptoms of heart illness can change depending on what's causing it.

Symptoms of irregular cardiac rhythms include, but are not limited to:

- a pounding or racing heart (palpitations).
- Aching in the chest
- Sweating.
- Lightheadedness.
- Uneasy and shallow breaths

symptoms of a disease that affects the heart valves.

- Dizziness
- Tiredness.
- Aching in the chest
- Heart murmur.
- Uneasy and shallow breaths

symptoms you experience if there is a blockage in the blood arteries in your heart, other organs, or anywhere else in your body.

- Pain in the chest or upper body
- An ache in the neck
- Indigestion or heartburn can be painful.

- Exhaustion.
- Uneasy and shallow breaths
- Nausea and/or vomiting may occur.
- Dizziness.

symptoms that might occur when your heart is having trouble pumping blood.

- Swelling in your lower body
- Exhaustion.
- Uneasy and shallow breaths

Heart conditions that you are born with may already present with symptoms, such as

- a heart murmur.
- Incapacity to deal with physical activity.
- Uneasy and shallow breath.

symptoms caused by problems with the lining of your heart.

- Chest discomfort that is often acute and is made worse when deep breathing is done
- Exhaustion.
- Having a hard time breathing
- You are experiencing swelling in your lower body.

It is essential to keep in mind that although women and older persons may exhibit less obvious symptoms, they may nonetheless be suffering from a severe form of cardiovascular disease.

Diagnosis And Tests

How exactly does one go about diagnosing cardiovascular disease?

Your doctor or other medical professional will conduct a physical exam and inquire about your symptoms, as well as your health and the medical history of your family. They might also request tests to assist in the diagnosis of cardiovascular disease if they deem it necessary.

What kinds of heart disease testing are available to me?

Some frequent tests to diagnose cardiovascular disease include:

- An examination of the patient's blood will measure chemicals in the blood that indicate the health of the cardiovascular system, such as cholesterol and certain proteins.
- An electrocardiogram, more commonly known as an EKG, is a test that monitors the electrical activity in your heart.
- In ambulatory monitoring, you wear monitors on your body that keep an eye on your heart rate and rhythm.
- The image of your heartbeat and blood flow that is produced by an echocardiogram is created by sound waves.

- X-rays are utilized in the cardiac CT procedure to produce images of the patient's heart and blood vessels.
- The images of your heart that are produced by cardiac MRI are created with the use of magnets and radio waves.
- EKGs and/or pictures are used in stress testing. These studies involve subjecting the heart to a regulated amount of stress in one of several different methods (exercise or drugs, for example), and then observing how the heart reacts.
- In cardiac catheterization, a catheter, which is a thin, hollow tube, is used to assess the pressure in your heart as well as the blood flow.

The management as well as treatment of cardiovascular disease

What kind of treatment is there for cardiovascular disease?

Treatment regimens can be different for each patient because they are based on the symptoms as well as the specific type of cardiovascular disease they have. Cardiovascular disease treatment may include:

1. **Alterations to one's lifestyle:** may include, for instance, making alterations to one's food, increasing the amount of aerobic activity one participates in, and giving up smoking.

2. **Medication:** To keep the cardiovascular disease under control, your healthcare practitioner may prescribe medication for you. The sort of cardiovascular illness you have will determine the medication that is prescribed to you.
3. In cases where the usage of drugs alone is not sufficient to control the symptoms of cardiovascular disease, your healthcare practitioner may recommend that you undergo specific surgical operations or other types of procedures to treat your condition. A few examples of these procedures are the implantation of stents in the coronary arteries of the heart or the legs, minimally invasive heart surgery, open-heart surgery, ablations, and cardioversion.
4. Rehabilitating your heart may require you to participate in an exercise program under supervision so that your heart can get stronger.
5. **Active surveillance:** If you do not take any medications or undergo any procedures or operations, you may need to be carefully monitored over time.

Will participating in cardiac rehabilitation make my treatment more effective?

Regaining strength in your heart is one of the goals of cardiac rehabilitation. It gives you additional assistance while you make changes to your lifestyle. It also includes exercise that is closely monitored and nutritional coaching.

If you require surgery on your heart, your doctor may suggest that you participate in cardiac rehabilitation. If you are recovering from a heart attack or stroke, you may also be eligible for rehabilitation services.

If you're having problems following the treatment plan that your cardiovascular disease prescribes for you on your own, cardiac rehabilitation is another option to consider. Inquire with your healthcare practitioner about your potential participation in a hospital-based program. They might advise you to participate in another program that is secure and beneficial to your health.

Prevention

How can I protect myself from developing heart disease?

Some forms of cardiovascular disease, such as congenital heart disease, cannot be avoided through preventative measures. Alterations to one's way of life, however, can cut one's risk of developing a variety of cardiovascular diseases.

Your risk of acquiring cardiovascular disease can be decreased by:

1. avoiding any goods containing tobacco.
2. dealing with additional health issues, such as diabetes, high cholesterol, or high blood pressure, and managing these problems effectively.
3. obtaining and keeping a healthy weight is the goal here.

4. Consuming a diet that is low in both salt and saturated fat.
5. Exercising for at least thirty to sixty minutes on most days of the week.
6. lowering and controlling one's stress levels.

Outlook / Prognosis

What is the prognosis for those who have been diagnosed with cardiovascular disease?

With the assistance of their healthcare team, a lot of people can keep their cardiovascular disease under control and still have a great quality of life. Participating actively in your healthcare and adhering to the treatment plan that you and your healthcare practitioner developed together will increase the likelihood that you will experience a favorable outcome. It is essential to take drugs precisely as directed by the doctor.

Do I have a higher chance of developing other problems if I have cardiovascular disease?

Cardiovascular illness that goes untreated can result in several significant problems.

If you suffer from cardiovascular disease, there is a possibility that you will have an increased risk of:

- Acute coronary syndrome
- Stroke.

- Acute limb ischemia (sudden blockage of the leg arteries).
- Dissection of the aorta
- Sudden cardiac death.

Living With It

When should I schedule my next visit with my primary care doctor?

When detected at an earlier stage, cardiovascular illness is typically easier for medical professionals to treat. You should make an appointment with your primary care physician as soon as possible if you see any symptoms of cardiovascular disease.

If you suddenly encounter any of the following, you should call 911 or seek emergency medical attention:

- Aching in the chest
- Convulsions (fainting).
- Extreme difficulty in breathing, particularly if it is recent or getting worse.
- You may be experiencing pain or numbness in your arms or legs.
- Ripping or tearing back discomfort.

Chapter 6

The Importance of Getting Enough Rest

A person must get adequate sleep to help them maintain their ideal level of health and well-being. Sleep is just as important to their overall health as maintaining a regular exercise routine and eating a nutritionally sound diet.

The contemporary style of life in the United States and many other nations does not often acknowledge the significance of getting sufficient amounts of sleep. Nevertheless, people need to make the effort to get enough sleep consistently.

The following is a short list of the numerous benefits that having adequate sleep is associated with, according to professionals in the medical field.

1. Increased efficiency and capacity for focused attention

Several research projects were carried out by medical professionals at the beginning of this century to investigate the impacts of inadequate sleep.

According to the findings of the study, sleep is linked to several different cognitive processes, including the following:

concentration\sproductivity\scognition

A more recent study, which was published in 2015 in the Journal of Child Psychology and Psychiatry, demonstrated that the sleeping patterns of children can have an indirect influence on the way they behave and how well they succeed in school.

2. Lower weight gain risk

The connection between insufficient sleep and increased risk of obesity and weight gain is not entirely understood.

Over the years, lots of research have established a connection between obesity and dysfunctional sleeping patterns.

On the other hand, a more recent study that was published in the journal Sleep Medicine concluded that there is no correlation between being overweight and not getting enough sleep.

According to the findings of this study, many of the earlier studies did not fully take into consideration additional characteristics such as:

- drinking alcohol
- levels of living with type 2 diabetes, levels of physical activity, and levels of education
- lengthy periods of employment followed by extended periods of inactivity
- A person's desire or capacity to maintain a healthy lifestyle may be negatively impacted by a lack of sleep, although sleep deprivation itself may or may not be a direct driver of weight gain.

3. Better calorie regulation

In a manner analogous to putting on weight, there is evidence to suggest that having an adequate amount of sleep each night can assist a person in consuming fewer calories throughout the day.

For instance, according to the findings of a study that was published in the Proceedings of the National Academy of Sciences of the United States of AmericaReliable Source, the patterns of sleep can influence the hormones that are responsible for appetite.

When a person does not sleep for the recommended amount of time, it can impair their body's capacity to effectively manage the amount of food they take in.

4. Improved success in athletic competition

The National Sleep Foundation recommends that individuals need between 7 and 9 hours of sleep per night, while athletes may benefit from getting as much as 10 hours of sleep. As a result, getting enough sleep is just as crucial for athletes as getting the proper amount of calories and nutrients.

The need for this is due, in part, to the fact that the body repairs itself while one is sleeping. Other advantages include the following:

increased levels of performance intensity

greater vitality, enhanced coordination, accelerated speed, and improved mental performance.

5. Reduced likelihood of developing heart disease

High blood pressure is one of the risk factors for cardiovascular disease. According to the Centers for Disease Control and Prevention (CDC), the ability of the body to manage one's blood pressure can be facilitated by receiving a suitable amount of sleep each night.

When this is done, there is a decreased risk of developing sleep-related problems such as apnea, and there is an improvement in the general health of the heart.

6. Greater intelligence in social and emotional situations

People's emotional and social intelligence may be affected by the amount of sleep they get. Someone who does not receive the recommended amount of sleep is more likely to have trouble understanding the feelings and expressions that other people are trying to convey.

For instance, research that was published in the Journal of Sleep Research (a peer-reviewed journal) looked at how people reacted to various emotional triggers. The researchers came to the conclusion, which is consistent with the findings of many other studies, that a person's capacity for emotional empathy is diminished when they do not obtain an acceptable amount of sleep.

7. Methods for avoiding mental illness

Research into the relationship between getting enough sleep and maintaining good mental health has been going on for quite some time. One possible interpretation is that there is a connection between insufficient sleep and feelings of depression.

Patterns of death by suicide were investigated over ten years in a study that was published in JAMA Psychiatry. It concludes that a lack of sleep is a contributing factor in many of these deaths.

People who have sleep disorders such as insomnia are more likely to display signs of depression, according to the findings of another study that was published in the Australian and New Zealand Journal of Psychiatry.

8. Reduce levels of inflammation

There is a correlation between obtaining enough sleep and having a reduced inflammatory response throughout the body.

For instance, a study that was published in the World Journal of Gastroenterology (a journal that is considered to be a reliable source) reveals that there may be a connection between lack of sleep and inflammatory bowel illnesses, which are conditions that damage people's digestive tracts.

According to the findings of the study, lack of sleep can play a role in the development of various diseases, and the diseases themselves can play a role in the development of sleep deprivation.

9. Stronger immune system

During sleep, the body can mend itself, renew, and recover. This link applies to everything, including the body's immune system. There is some evidence that a higher quality of sleep can assist the body in its battle against infection.

However, to fully understand how sleep affects the immune system of the body, scientists still need to do additional research into the specific mechanisms involved.

Sleep suggestions

The amount of sleep that an individual need changes significantly with age. The amount of sleep a person normally needs to operate properly decreases as they become older.

The following is the distribution, as reported by the CDC:

- 14–17 hours for newborns (ages 0–3 months).
- Newborns (4–12 months): between 12 and 16 hours
- 11–14 hours for a toddler (1–2 years old)
- 10–13 hours each day for children ages 3–5 in preschool.
- Children in school (ages 6 to 12): nine to twelve hours
- Teenagers (ages 13–18): eight to ten hours
- Adults (18–60 years old): seven hours or more
- Adults (ages 61–64): seven to nine hours
- 7–8 hours for adults (those aged 65 and up).

It is not enough to simply get enough hours of sleep; the quality of that sleep is also essential. Some of the following are symptoms of poor sleep quality:

Despite having gotten the required amount of sleep, I do not feel refreshed in the morning.

The following are some of the things a person can do to improve the quality of their sleep:

- Avoid going back to sleep after you've already received enough rest for the night.
- Increasing the amount of time spent outside and the amount of physical activity performed during the day.
- stress reduction achieved through physical activity, psychotherapy, or other techniques.

In conclusion, sleep is essential, although frequently disregarded component of the total health and well-being of every individual. Because it allows the body to mend itself and get itself ready for the next day, sleep is critically necessary.

It has been suggested that getting a proper amount of rest can also assist avoid the accumulation of excess weight, heart disease, and an extended period of illness.

Chapter 7

Consuming foods that promote longevity and health

According to the findings of numerous scientific studies, there is a correlation between eating well and living a longer and better life.

But for a variety of reasons, getting older might make it more challenging for some people to maintain a healthy diet. Perhaps they don't have much of an appetite at the moment. They may have problems preparing food or eating. Perhaps they are unaware of what constitutes a healthy lifestyle. Or perhaps they do, but they just don't like the flavor of kale.
"Do you realize what? According to Cheryl Rock, Ph.D., a professor of family medicine and public health at the University of California, San Diego School of Medicine, "You may live a long and healthy life without ever eating a slice of kale," and she is right.

She is an advocate for locating nutritious foods that one enjoys eating and expanding on that foundation.

If you're eating things that you enjoy, you'll have a better chance of sticking with your diet. Rock predicts that you won't be able to push it down for four days and then reward yourself with a double cheeseburger.

However, selecting the appropriate foods is only part of the challenge. In addition, as Michele Bellantoni of the Johns Hopkins University School of Medicine points out, it is important to consume them in the appropriate quantities.
According to her, "it appears that the best number of calories [for the majority of older persons] will be 1,800 [per day]." And to age healthily, we must consider instead of concentrating on certain body parts, consider the entire body.

There are a lot of meals that are particularly beneficial to various regions of your body. Bellantoni recommends allocating those 1,800 calories to get adequate amounts of protein for your muscles, calcium for your bones, and a diet that is generally good for your heart.

This tactic could let you access a lot of opportunities.

It may be beneficial to your heart

Your weight control can benefit from adopting a diet that is good for your heart. This is significant given that a greater than one-third of adults aged 65 and older are overweight. Diabetes, some malignancies, and heart disease are all potential outcomes of this.
A diet that is healthy for the heart contains foods such as:

- Fruits and vegetables
- Whole grains
- yogurt and cheese are examples of low-fat dairy products.
- Poultry without a skin
- A great deal of fish
- Almonds and kidney beans
- oils from plants grown outside of the tropics (olive, corn, peanut, and safflower oils)
- Omega-3 fatty acids are found in high concentrations in some fish, such as salmon, trout, and herring. These acids help reduce the risk of developing heart disease and may also be beneficial for those who suffer from high blood pressure. Aim for two servings per week as a general rule.

It may be beneficial to your brain

Several factors have been connected to a deficiency of vitamin B12, one of which is memory loss, which is a major worry among certain older persons. That is available in
Vegetables and Fruits
Products made from fish milk
A few Options for Breakfast Cereals
There is a connection between Alzheimer's disease and chronic inflammation, which can be brought on by eating certain foods including white bread, french fries, red meat, sugary beverages, and margarine.

The relationship between the consumption of certain meals and the health of the brain is still being investigated by scientists.

"I would not want to single out a certain kind of meal as the one that helps prevent memory loss. According to Adam Drewnowski, Ph.D., "If you want to be operating well, some fruits and antioxidants will do better for you than another slice of cake." director of the Nutritional Sciences Program at the University of Washington. I would probably advise someone that eating fruits and antioxidants will benefit them more than eating another piece of cake if they want to be operating effectively.
Antioxidants, which can be found in blueberries and other fruits and vegetables, are known to help reduce inflammation. They also assist you in getting rid of potentially harmful substances known as free radicals, which are produced

whenever your body converts the fuel you eat into usable energy.

Again, it is essential to keep in mind that maintaining excellent brain health may depend on what you avoid eating just as much as it does on what you do consume.
According to Rock, "your brain runs on blood flow, much like your heart," which is an interesting observation. Therefore, consuming a diet high in saturated fats makes it less likely that a person will have the good, clean arteries necessary to deliver blood to the brain tissue.

Make it a point to include in your diet things like tomatoes, blueberries, dark green leafy vegetables like spinach and kale, turmeric, and nuts, particularly walnuts. In addition, the omega-3 fatty acids that can be found in salmon and other oily fish are effective in reducing inflammation.

It Might Be Beneficial to Your Muscles

They are always being broken down and then getting built back up again since that is the way that your body functions. As you get older, your body's demand for protein to assist in the process of rebuilding increases.

According to Rock, if you don't get enough protein in your diet, you'll end up degrading your muscles more quickly than you can rebuild them.

Beans, lean meats, fish, and other types of seafood, yogurt, cheese, and milk that are low in fat or fat-free, and cheese and milk are all dairy products. Additionally, eggs are a fantastic source of protein, and in contrast to meat, they do not include any saturated fats in their composition. According to Rock, you shouldn't be concerned about the amount of cholesterol in your eggs. Your body doesn't absorb it well.

It May Be Beneficial to Your Bones

Calcium is essential for the growth and maintenance of strong bones in older persons. Milk, yogurt, and cheeses with low-fat content are all good sources.

However, you should exercise caution because consuming an excessive amount can lead to constipation. Have a conversation about what's best for you with your primary care physician or a dietician.

Consuming an adequate amount of vitamin D is also essential since this vitamin facilitates the absorption of calcium in the body. But accomplishing that isn't always simple. According to Stephen Anton, Ph.D., from the department of aging and geriatric research at the University of Florida, "the risk for low vitamin D in older folks, it's sort of an issue because it's not like there are tons of foods that are high in vitamin D."

Fortified meals, fatty fish such as salmon, and dairy products are good sources of calcium and vitamin D.

Chapter 8

The Many Advantages of Exercise

The term "exercise" refers to any physical activity that compels your muscles to contract and forces your body to use up calories in the process.

There are many different kinds of physical activities, some examples of which are dancing, walking, running, and jogging. Swimming is another popular choice.

Research has proven that being active has many positive effects on one's health, both physically and emotionally. It might help you live for a longer time.

The following are the top ten ways that your body and brain benefit from frequent exercise.

1. Physical activity has the potential to improve one's mood.

Exercising can help boost your mood and reduce feelings of despair, worry, and stress, according to several studies.

It causes alterations in the regions of the brain that are responsible for regulating anxiety and stress. Additionally, it has the potential to boost the brain's sensitivity to the neurotransmitters serotonin and norepinephrine, both of which work to alleviate the symptoms of depression.

Endorphins are known to assist promote happy feelings and lower the impression of pain. Exercise can help enhance the production of endorphins, which can help lessen the experience of pain.

It is interesting to note that the intensity of your workout does not make a difference. It would appear that the benefits of exercise on mood are unrelated to the level of intensity of the physical activity.

According to the findings of a study conducted on a group of 24 women who had been clinically diagnosed with depression, any level of physical activity dramatically reduced feelings of depression.

The effects of exercise on mood are so potent that the decision to exercise (or not exercise) even makes a difference over very short periods.

After only a few weeks, inactive adults who stopped exercising regularly reported significant increases in feelings of despair and anxiety, according to the findings of a study of 19 separate studies on the topic.

2. Participating in physical activity can facilitate weight loss.

According to the findings of several studies, one of the primary contributors to weight gain and obesity is a sedentary lifestyle.

It is essential to have an understanding of the connection between physical activity and the number of calories burned to comprehend the impact that exercise has on weight loss (spending).

Through exercise, you may ensure that your body's processes, such as your heartbeat and breathing, continue uninterrupted. If you limit the number of calories you consume while dieting, your metabolic rate will decrease, which may momentarily slow down your weight loss. On the other hand, it has been demonstrated that engaging in regular physical activity can boost your metabolism, leading to an increase in the number of calories burned during the day.

In addition, studies have shown that combining aerobic exercise with resistance training will maximize fat loss and retain muscle mass, which is critical for preserving lean muscle mass and not regaining weight after weight reduction.

3. Regular exercise is beneficial to the health of both your muscles and bones.

The development and upkeep of strong muscles and bones are both significantly aided by regular exercise.

When combined with a sufficient diet of protein, resistance training activities like weightlifting can help drive muscle growth.

Because it helps release hormones that improve your muscles' ability to absorb amino acids, exercise is a key factor in this phenomenon. This encourages their growth and minimizes the risk of their breaking down.

People tend to lose both muscle mass and function as they become older, which might put them at a greater risk of being injured. It is necessary to engage in regular physical activity if you want to slow the atrophy of your muscles and keep your strength as you become older.

In addition to assisting in the prevention of osteoporosis in later years, exercise can also assist in the development of healthy bone density in younger individuals.

Some studies suggest that activities with a high impact, such as gymnastics or running, or sports with an unusually high impact, such as soccer and basketball, may assist develop a higher bone density than activities with no impact, such as swimming and cycling.

4. Physical activity has been shown to boost one's energy levels

For many people, including those with a variety of medical issues, physical activity can be a significant boost to their energy levels.

An older study indicated that 36 participants who had reported continuous exhaustion experienced a reduction in sensations of fatigue after participating in regular exercise for six weeks.

A healthy heart and lungs are two of the many wonderful benefits that come from regular physical activity. Aerobic exercise enhances both the cardiovascular system and the health of the lungs, both of which can contribute significantly to an individual's overall energy levels.

When you walk around more, your heart pumps more blood, which brings more oxygen to the muscles that are actively working. Your muscles will become more efficient as a result of your heart becoming more effective and skilled at delivering oxygen into your blood if you continue to exercise regularly.

This aerobic training over time results in less strain being placed on your lungs, as well as less energy being required to do the same tasks. This is one of the reasons why you are less likely to experience chest pain or dizziness when engaging in strenuous activity.

In addition to this, research has shown that patients with various disorders, such as cancer, have higher energy levels after engaging in physical activity.

5. Regular exercise lowers the risk of developing chronic diseases

One of the key contributors to the development of chronic disease is a sedentary lifestyle.

It has been demonstrated that engaging in consistent physical activity can enhance insulin sensitivity, cardiovascular health, and body composition. Additionally, it has the potential to lower both blood pressure and cholesterol levels.

To be more specific, physical activity can assist in the reduction or prevention of the following persistent health conditions:

Type 2 diabetes. Type 2 diabetes may be delayed or prevented with regular aerobic exercise. People who have type 1 diabetes can also reap significant health benefits from consuming it. The benefits of resistance training for type 2 diabetes include reductions in fat mass, reductions in blood pressure, increases in lean body mass, and improvements in insulin resistance and glycemic management.

Coronary artery disease People who already suffer from cardiovascular disease can benefit from exercise not just as a preventative measure but also as a treatment.

There are numerous forms of cancer. Exercising regularly can assist in lowering one's chance of developing many different types of cancer, including breast, colorectal, endometrial, gallbladder, kidney, lung, liver, ovarian, pancreatic, prostate, thyroid, gastric, and esophageal cancer.

Poor cholesterol levels. Regular physical activity of moderate intensity can raise HDL cholesterol (the "good" cholesterol), while also preserving or balancing increases in LDL cholesterol (the "bad" cholesterol). The hypothesis that high-intensity aerobic activity is necessary to lower LDL levels is supported by research to some extent.

Hypertension: Regular participation in aerobic exercise can reduce resting systolic blood pressure by 5–7 millimeters of mercury in those who have hypertension.

On the other hand, a lack of consistent physical activity — even for a very short period — can lead to considerable increases in abdominal fat, which in turn may increase the risk of type 2 diabetes and heart disease.

Because of this, it is advisable to engage in regular physical activity to lower the amount of abdominal fat and the risk of getting these illnesses.

6. Regular exercise is good for the health of your skin

The level of oxidative stress that is present in your body has the potential to affect your skin.

The condition known as oxidative stress happens when the antioxidant defenses of the body are unable to properly repair the cell damage caused by molecules known as free radicals. This can cause the structure of the cells to become compromised, which will have a bad effect on your skin.

Even though strenuous and intensive physical activity might add to oxidative damage, regular moderate exercise can improve your body's production of natural antioxidants, which can assist in protecting cells from harm caused by free radicals.

Similarly, physical activity can increase blood flow and cause changes in skin cells, both of which can help delay the visible signs of aging in the skin.

7. Regular exercise can improve both the health of your brain and your memory.

Physical activity has been shown to boost brain function, as well as safeguard memory and thinking abilities.

To begin, it raises your heart rate, which in turn increases the amount of blood and oxygen that is being delivered to your brain. In addition to this, it has the potential to increase the production of hormones that promote the expansion of brain cells.

In addition, the capacity of exercise to avoid chronic disease can translate into benefits for your brain, as the function of your brain can be impacted by conditions such as these.

It is especially crucial for older persons to engage in regular physical activity since the natural process of aging when combined with oxidative stress and inflammation, causes changes in the brain's structure and function.

It has been demonstrated that regular exercise can cause the hippocampus, a region of the brain that is essential for memory and learning, to enlarge, which may contribute to an improvement in cognitive performance in older adults.

Last but not least, research has revealed that regular exercise helps mitigate changes in the brain that are associated with the development of Alzheimer's disease and dementia.

8. Regular exercise can facilitate relaxation and improve the quality of sleep

Your ability to relax and get a better night's sleep may improve if you exercise regularly.

When it comes to the quality of sleep, the depletion (loss) of energy that takes place during exercise stimulates the restorative processes that take place during sleep.

Additionally, the rise in core body temperature that accompanies physical activity is thought to improve the quality of sleep by assisting in the reduction of core body temperature when one is asleep.

There have been lots of research done on the effects of exercise on sleep, and all of them have come to the same results.

Participation in an exercise training program was found to assist enhance self-reported sleep quality as well as reduce sleep latency, which is the amount of time it takes to fall asleep. These findings were obtained in a review of six separate research.

People who had chronic insomnia benefited from both stretching and resistance training, according to the findings of a study that was carried out over four months.

Stretching and strength training both led to improvements in the ability to fall back asleep after waking up, as well as in the length and quality of sleep that resulted. The stretching group saw a reduction in anxious feelings as well.

In addition, research suggests that older persons, who are frequently plagued by sleep difficulties, may benefit from engaging in regular physical activity.

You have some leeway in terms of the type of physical activity that you pick. It would suggest that either aerobic exercise on its own or aerobic exercise in conjunction with resistance training can improve the quality of sleep.

9. Exercise can reduce pain

Exercising, even though chronic pain can be incapacitating at times, can help reduce the pain.

In point of fact, for a considerable amount of time, the advice given to treat chronic pain was to remain inactive and to get plenty of rest. Recent research, on the other hand, suggests that physical activity can help alleviate chronic pain.

One study that analyzed the findings of several others discovered that exercise can help people who suffer from chronic pain reduce their pain and improve their quality of life.

Exercise has also been shown in several studies to be effective in the management of pain associated with a variety of health disorders. These conditions include chronic low back pain, fibromyalgia, and chronic soft tissue shoulder disorder, to name just a few.

In addition, physical activity can both increase a person's pain tolerance and diminish their ability to feel pain.

10. Regular physical activity can contribute to an improved sexual life.

Exercising regularly has been shown to increase sexual desire.

Regular exercise can improve your sex life in several ways, including strengthening the heart, enhancing blood circulation, toning muscles, and increasing flexibility.

In addition to enhancing sexual performance and sexual enjoyment, regular physical activity can also increase the amount of time spent engaging in sexual activity.
In a study involving 405 postmenopausal women, it was shown that regular exercise was connected with increased sexual function and desire. This finding is quite interesting.

An evaluation of ten separate research concluded that engaging in physical activity for at least six months at a time for a minimum of 160 minutes per week was associated with a noticeable rise in the level of erection success experienced by males.

In addition, a different study indicated that a straightforward routine consisting of a 6-minute walk around the house helped 41 men experience a 71% reduction in the severity of their erectile dysfunction symptoms.

Another study found that women with polycystic ovary syndrome, a condition that can cause a decrease in sexual desire, were able to enhance their sex drive by engaging in regular resistance training for 16 weeks.
In a nutshell, physical activity confers a plethora of advantageous effects, nearly all of which are beneficial to one's overall health. The synthesis of hormones that make you feel happy and help you sleep better can be increased by engaging in physical activity regularly.

Additionally, it can:

Enhance the overall appearance of your skin.
assist you in achieving and maintaining a healthy weight, hence lowering your risk of developing chronic diseases.
Enhance your sexual experience.
In addition, you don't need to do a lot of exercises for it to have a significant impact on your health.

You will comply with the Department of Health and Human Services' activity guidelines for adults if you set a weekly goal of between 150 and 300 minutes of aerobic activity with moderate intensity or 75 minutes of strenuous physical activity spread out over the week.

Walking, cycling, and swimming are examples of activities that fall into the category of having an aerobic effort level that is considered to be moderate. Running or taking part in a physically demanding exercise class are examples of activities that qualify as vigorous intensity.

You will exceed the requirements if you include at least two days of muscle-strengthening activities that involve all main muscle groups (legs, hips, back abdomen, chest, shoulders, and arms).

Strengthening your muscles can be accomplished by the use of free weights, resistance bands, or even just your body weight. Squats, push-ups, shoulder presses, chest presses, and planks are some examples of these exercises.

You may invariably enhance your health in a variety of ways, regardless of whether you participate in a particular sport or adhere to the recommendation of engaging in physical exercise for a total of two hours and thirty minutes every week

Why physical activity doesn't have to make you hot and uncomfortable

The majority of people believe that a good workout causes them to break out in a sweat. They do not believe they have achieved their goals until they are completely drenched in their sweat. But should we think of sweating as a useful indicator of how hard we worked out? After a very strenuous workout, some people don't even break a sweat. The warm temperature of the environment might also cause a person to sweat. It is therefore not accurate to evaluate the effectiveness of your workout primarily on the amount of perspiration that you produce.

How to evaluate the effectiveness of your work

Believe us when we say that being drenched in sweat does not indicate a successful workout. To get the most out of your workout, you need to push yourself to your limitations. You shouldn't stick to your normal training routine and should instead try new things every time you work out. It is acceptable even if you only make a little bit of headway. When you leave the gym, your goal shouldn't be to be drenched in sweat but rather to have accomplished your goal for the session and to feel better. Only after the intended purpose of the session is accomplished can one consider the workout to have been successful.

Is it significant that you sweat?

No, it is not necessary to break a sweat during each one of your workouts at the gym. It is not possible to evaluate a person's productivity simply on the amount of sweat that they have produced. Because of their genes, some people tend to sweat more than others. In addition, people tend to not sweat as much during a session of strength training since their heart rate does not get as elevated as it does during a session of cardiovascular exercise. That doesn't mean they aren't putting in a lot of effort, though.

Some individuals even continue to perform the same exercises over and over again to guarantee that they will break a nice sweat. However, doing so is not going to be of much value to them since it may result in overtraining and a halt in their weight loss.

The bare essentials

The amount of sweat that you produce is determined by several different factors, including your genetics, degree of hydration, and surroundings. It has very little bearing on the effectiveness of what you accomplish. Therefore, you shouldn't evaluate your fitness level primarily on how much sweat you produce during physical activity. Continue to push yourself beyond your comfort zone and incorporate new exercises into your everyday regimen.

Chapter 9

Increase your level of physical fitness and monitor your improvement

You decide to make exercise a priority. You put in some time at the gym over multiple days. You give up on your goals after a week or two of not seeing any progress, which is why you set them. (We've been there.) Time passes. You decide to start working out again. Repeat.

Put an end to this cycle!

Progress doesn't happen overnight. It takes time and effort before one may see benefits. Keeping a record of your achievements along the road is the most effective method for achieving your fitness objectives.

Alterations in both your physical state and the way you feel are wonderful motivators for movement. Monitoring your advancement not only boosts the probability that you'll achieve your objective but also pushes you to make the most of the time you have available. When you find that you can do more reps than you could the last time or that your clothes fit differently, you'll want to keep pushing forward with your routine.

How can you tell if the change you're trying to make is happening? Investigate the eight methods listed here for measuring your development in fitness. It's possible that you won't know what works best for you till you try a few different things.

1. Maintain a Health and Fitness Journal.

Keeping a journal is a straightforward method that can be utilized to monitor one's progression. It is not necessary to overcomplicate the process of keeping track of your exercises and meals. You can use a paper notepad and a pen, the digital notes feature on your iPhone, or a spreadsheet created in Excel.

Put in writing the exercises you did and the number of sets or repetitions you completed. Make a note of the weight that you used for any strengthening exercises that you did. Record the time that you ran the mile if you did it. Include how you feel after the workout in your post-workout reflection. How difficult were the exercises, or how easy were they? Do you feel energized?

Your journal is an excellent location for keeping a record of your diet as well. Exercise on its own won't get you the results you want or make you feel more confident in your skin. In addition to it, a healthy diet is required.

Extreme measures must be taken if one is going to count calories for everything, every day. We suggest keeping a food journal for at least a week to have a better understanding of your eating habits. If you pay attention to your eating patterns, you'll be able to see if you're not getting enough wholesome, nutritious foods or if you're snacking on an excessive amount of potato chips between lunch and supper.

Use this opportunity to educate yourself about what you now eat and how much of it you consume. The next step is to seek out opportunities to eat healthier meals or more modest portions.

2. Make use of a fitness tracker or mobile application

Letting technology take the lead in monitoring one's fitness development is yet another method. Apps, smartwatches, and fitness trackers all display and retain the useful data that is generated by your workouts. You can track your heart rate over time with an Apple Watch or a Fitbit, and it will tell you exactly how many steps you've taken over the day.

You have the option to use more conventional methods if you are keeping track of your steps. A pedometer that does not have a lot of other features but counts your steps is sufficient.

There are a lot of applications out there that can help you track your fitness progress.

MyFitnessPal gives you the tools you need to make healthy decisions for yourself. On the app, you can plan meals, as well as log meals, establish nutrition goals, and use nutritional insights.

You may use FitNotes to keep track of your movement whether you're at home or in the gym. Include the following information in your workout logs: repetitions, distances, and times.

Strongly is another app that tracks your workouts and your fitness. You can keep track of your prior exercises and plan out your future fitness regimens using Strongly. This software keeps track of the overall mass moved throughout each workout.

Jefit enables you to create individualized workouts and make preparations for your next session. You can keep track of your workouts, concentrate on your body statistics, and evaluate your progress as you go.

3. Take Pictures of Your Workout Progress.

Bring on the selfies once you've finished your workout! Our perception of our bodies shifts throughout the day as a result of the constant exposure to the mirror. It's not always easy to keep track of all how you've improved over time. You will be able to see the changes in your body from week one to week eight through the use of progress images.

Make it a point to take images of your progress from the same angles, at the same time of day, and in the same light. Since your weight changes during the day, a picture of you taken when you first wake up and one taken after you've eaten will appear to be very different from one another. The way your physique appears in an image is also impacted by the lighting. Poor lighting might cause shadows, which can disguise your progress and slow you down. Taking pictures of your progress while wearing the same outfit or outfits that are identical to one another lets you identify the differences more easily.

After you have taken the photographs, put them away somewhere safe for later use. Do not evaluate the current images based on those taken three days ago. You want to look at images that were taken between four and six weeks apart from each other.

4. Observe the sizing of your garments.

Utilizing your wardrobe as a gauge for your improvement is a useful strategy. Locate the shirt you wish to fill out and put it on. Bring the pair of jeans you'd like to be able to wear again into the room.

The way an article of clothing fits can be used as a barometer to determine whether or not you are making progress toward your objectives. Does the outfit appear to be more relaxed? Tighter? If you decide to utilize a piece of clothing as a way to motivate yourself, we suggest picking out the same article of clothing and monitoring your progress once a month.

5. Step on the Scale

The scale is frequently the method of choice when attempting to quantify a weight decrease. However, the scale is not going to tell you the whole truth about your weight. The factors responsible for daily shifts in weight are water retention and bowel movement. Your body will retain water if you consume foods high in sodium, vegetables, and soups that are high in water content, excessive amounts of carbohydrates, and alcohol.

The average daily weight change for an adult is between two and six pounds. It is common for one's weight to fluctuate daily. They won't be able to prevent you from reaching your objectives in any way. Be on the lookout for increases in weight that are significant and continue for more than a day or two. These increases are not the result of an increase in water content; nevertheless, they may indicate that you are gaining muscle.

If the number on the scale is everything to you, we suggest limiting your weighing to once a week and utilizing other metrics in addition to the scale to monitor your progress. After you've used the restroom and gotten dressed in the morning, go on the scale.

6. Take Measurements

The fact that muscle weighs more than fat is one of the reasons why a scale can be misleading. Because it is more lean than fat, your muscle takes up less room in your body. When you measure your physique, you will notice that it has changed in small increments.

As is the case with the scale, we do not advise measuring every day. Once a week or once every other week, measure your neck, shoulders, chest, biceps, waist, hips, and thighs with a tape measure to keep track of your progress. When taking your measurements, use the same conditions and time of day each time.

Calculating your waist-to-hip ratio can provide you with a more comprehensive measurement if that's what you're looking for. This ratio provides you with a general notion of how healthy you are overall.

Measure your waist as well as your hips. After that, divide the circumference of your hips by the circumference of your waist. The final score should be 0.85 or below for women, and 0.9 or lower for men; anything greater than that indicates an elevated risk of cardiovascular disease and other chronic illnesses.

7. Perform a test of your squat.

Squatting is a great exercise to test both your core and leg strength. You should be standing with your feet about shoulder-width apart and your arms out in front of you in a straight line. If so, squat down! How does it feel? Are you able to do several squats while maintaining proper form? Do the insides of your knees cave inward? Do you have a stronger preference for one side over the other?

You might find it helpful to perform your squats in front of a mirror so that you can better monitor your form. Keep a close eye on both your front and your side at all times. Your technique will become better with practice, and you'll experience an increase in physical strength.

8. Have your blood pressure checked regularly.

There is more to progress than just making things seem nice. Your blood pressure gives you an accurate portrayal of your overall health and can help you determine whether you should focus on losing weight or gaining muscle first.

The degree to which exercise, nutrition, and stress all have a role in one's blood pressure is a useful predictor of one's heart health. Your body and your cardiovascular system become more robust as you continue to engage in increasingly strenuous physical activity. Your blood pressure may indicate a lower risk of heart disease and other chronic conditions.

9. Put Your Body Through Its Paces

The most important indicator of your level of development is how you feel. By putting your body through rigorous exercise, you may gauge your level of improved strength, flexibility, and endurance.

Choose an activity and make it a regular part of your routine. Are you able to increase the number of reps you performed compared to the previous month? Are you able to add weight? Does it appear that the workout is getting easier? When you track your progress in this manner, the focus is not on how your body appears but rather on what it is capable of doing.

The following are some examples:

- Plank. Every week, add a few more seconds. How long are you able to hold a plank for?
- Push-ups. Every week, add one additional rep to the total. Are you able to perform one additional push-up compared to the previous week?
- Burpees. Every week, add one additional rep to your total. Do the reps grow easier as you progress?

Your challenge could be something more significant, such as participating in a 5K race or signing up for a spin class regularly. You can gauge your overall improvement from one year to the next by keeping track of whether or not the aforementioned activities feel simpler or more challenging to complete. Have you improved upon your 5K time from the previous year? Did you run more than you walked? Challenge your body by including activities that you enjoy in your life.

10. Keep track of your active minutes

The third method for gauging one's improvement in fitness is to keep track of the number of minutes spent moving. We are aware that we need to keep moving for a minimum of half an hour, five days a week. If you want to be more active, counting minutes is an easy technique to help you add movement to your day. This should be your objective if you want to be more active.

The amount of time you spend being active daily can be monitored through fitness trackers and mobile applications. The müüv app monitors your progress in terms of minutes while also guiding you through various workout routines and intervals. The app will remember the total amount of time you spent moving once you finish an exercise, regardless of whether it was stretching, walking, or rowing.

There are a variety of techniques to keep track of your progress in terms of physical fitness. Depending on your lifestyle, personality, and the things you want to do, one strategy can work better for you than the other. You will be more motivated to continue working out and getting closer to the results you want to see if you keep track of your progress.

Chapter 10

The importance of muscular power for a long life

According to the lead researcher, Kate Duchowny, who just recently finished her doctorate in epidemiology at the University of Michigan School of Public Health, keeping one's muscle strength throughout one's entire life, and especially in later life, is extremely important for both living a long life and aging independently.

According to Duchowny, an expanding body of studies suggests that the strength of a person's muscles may be an even better indicator of overall health and lifespan than the amount of muscular mass they have.

It has also been discovered that mobility constraints and impairment have an inverse relationship with hand grip strength specifically. According to Duchowny, however, the measurement of grip strength is not currently included in the majority of regular physicals, even though it is a reasonably easy and cost-effective test.

According to Duchowny, who is currently doing postdoctoral research at the University of California, San Francisco, "This study further underlines the necessity of integrating grip strength assessments into routine care—not just for older persons but also in midlife." The evaluation of hand grip strength should be an essential element of normal medical care since it would make it possible to begin treatment at an earlier stage, which could result in persons living longer and enjoying greater levels of autonomy.

Data from a nationally representative sample of 8,326 men and women aged 65 and older who are participants in the Health and Retirement Study at the University of Michigan were evaluated by Duchowny and colleagues.

A device known as a dynamometer can be used to evaluate grip strength. This equipment requires the patient to squeeze it to determine their strength in kilograms. The researchers defined the different levels of strength by using "cut-points," also known as thresholds. For instance, having a hand grip strength of fewer than 39 kilograms for males or 22 kilograms for women was considered to be indicative of muscle weakness.

According to Duchowny, those thresholds were established using the nationally representative sample, which is exclusive to this study, according to Duchowny.

According to the findings, 46% of the sample population was assessed to be weak when compared to the baseline. In comparison, when considering other cut-points that were determined from samples with less representation, only roughly 10 to 13 percent of the samples were deemed to be poor.

"We feel our cut-points more accurately reflect the changing population patterns of older Americans and that muscle weakness is a critical public health concern," Duchowny said. "We believe our cut-points are more appropriate because they reflect the changing population trends of older Americans." "A significant number of studies on aging, including those that focus on measures of muscle strength, are carried out on primarily white populations. However, since the demographic makeup of the United States continues to shift, it is more important than ever to conduct research of this kind using data that is nationally representative

www.ingramcontent.com/pod-product-compliance
Lightning Source LLC
LaVergne TN
LVHW050330160826
845677LV00014B/3574

* 9 7 9 8 8 4 4 2 2 2 4 1 2 *